How Hospitals Survived

How Hospitals Survived

Competition and the American Hospital

David Dranove and
William D. White

The AEI Press

Publisher for the American Enterprise Institute

WASHINGTON, D.C.

1999

We would like to thank Mark Botti, Barry Harris, Robert Helms, Karl Kronebusch, two anonymous referees, and participants at the presentation of this work at the American Enterprise Institute's health policy discussion on December 4, 1998, for their comments. Any errors that remain are our own.

To order call toll free 1-800-462-6420 or 1-717-794-3800. For all other inquiries please contact the AEI Press, 1150 Seventeenth Street, N.W., Washington, D.C. 20036 or call 1-800-862-5801.

ISBN 978-0-8447-7141-0
ISBN 0-8447-7141-4

1 3 5 7 9 10 8 6 4 2

THE AEI PRESS
Publisher for the American Enterprise Institute
1150 Seventeenth Street, N.W.
Washington, D.C. 20036

Contents

1

Introduction

"The hospital is the core institutional provider of health care. Yet, for the reasons that follow, as their costs increase, hospitals will be in an increasingly vulnerable position within the health care market." Jeff C. Goldsmith, "The Health Care Market: Can Hospitals Survive?" *Harvard Business Review,* vol. 58, September–October 1980, pp. 100–112.

"The reports of my death are greatly exaggerated." Mark Twain, Cable from London to the Associated Press, 1897; in John Bartlett, *Familiar Quotations,* 13th ed. (New York: Little, Brown, 1955).

The modern hospital has its genesis in the early decades of the twentieth century. Until the end of the nineteenth century, the business of medicine was carried out almost entirely in doctors' offices and patients' homes. Hospital care was a small component of total healthcare spending. As late as 1870, a national survey identified fewer than 200 hospitals in the United States (White 1982). These hospitals were primarily vendors of last resort. They served patients who had nowhere else to turn—the indigent and those without friends or family. These patients usually could not afford to pay for care. Patients who had the means to do so typically went elsewhere, and most hospital revenue came from public funds and private charity.

The role of hospitals changed dramatically in the years around World War I (Stevens 1989). Advances in surgery, new diagnostic techniques, and social changes combined to make hospital care increasingly attractive to paying patients. In response to rising demand, hospitals began to serve a greatly expanded clientele and entry into the industry increased dramatically. Typically, newly established hospitals served their local communities and offered a wide range of disparate diagnostic and therapeutic inpatient services under one roof—hence the name "community general hospitals" or, for short, "community hospitals." By the late 1920s, there were more than 4,000 community hospitals with more than 300,000 beds in the United States. In 1929, as shown in table 1–1, hospital services accounted for some 20 percent of healthcare spending and .7 percent of the gross domestic product (White 1982; National Center for Health Statistics 1998).

By 1950, the community hospital was firmly established as the core institutional provider of medical care in the U.S. medical system. It had become the "doctor's workshop," giving physicians the equipment and nursing support necessary to offer a full range of acute care inpatient services in a single, centralized location. The growth of private health insurance following World War II and the introduction of Medicare and Medicaid in 1965 further fueled hospital growth. In 1975 there were almost 6,000 nonfederal hospitals in the United States, with nearly 950,000 beds. Hospital expenditures had risen to more than 40 percent of healthcare spending and accounted for 3.2 percent of the gross domestic product (National Center for Health Statistics 1998; American Hospital Association 1976).

The number of community hospital beds continued to grow until 1985, peaking at slightly over 1 million beds. By the end of the 1970s, however, healthcare industry experts such as Jeff Goldsmith were already posing the

TABLE 1-1
Spending on Hospital Care, All Hospitals, 1929–1996

Year	National Health Expenditures (billions)	National Health Expenditures as Percentage of Gross Domestic Product	Hospital Expenditures (billions)	Hospital Expenditures as Percentage of National Healthcare Expenditures	Hospital Expenditures as Percentage of Gross Domestic Product [a]
1929	3.6	3.5	0.7	19.4	0.7
1948	10.6	4.1	3.2	30.2	1.2
1955	17.7	4.4	5.9	33.3	1.5
1965	41.1	5.7	14.0	34.1	1.9
1975	130.7	8.0	52.6	40.2	3.2
1985	428.7	10.3	168.3	39.3	4.0
1996	1,035.1	13.6	358.5	34.6	4.7

a. For 1929, 1948, and 1955, percentages are reported as a share of gross national product.
SOURCES: 1929–1955: U.S. Bureau of the Census, *Historical Statistics of the United States, Colonial Times to 1970, Bicentennial Edition, Part 1* (Washington, D.C.: 1975); 1965–1996: National Center for Health Statistics, *Health, United States 1998* DHHS Publication (PHS) 98-1232, 1998.

question, "Will hospitals survive?" No one seriously argued that hospitals would vanish. But many raised questions about their future in the face of mounting healthcare expenditures and a shift toward market-oriented policies to contain costs. In particular, Goldsmith (1980, 1981) and others argued that the growth of outpatient surgery, home healthcare, freestanding imaging centers, and other outpatient services could relegate hospitals to a significantly diminished role as the specialized providers of high-end care.

Almost twenty years later, it is clear that these pessimistic predictions were premature. Hospitals remain the core institutional providers of care. In 1996 hospital expenditures still accounted for 35 percent of total healthcare spending. Perhaps more significant, their share of national income has increased to 4.7 percent (National Center for Health Statistics 1998). In absolute terms, hospitals are thus more important than ever before.

At the same time, the hospital of today looks quite different from the hospital of 1980, let alone 1950. Today's hospital offers a wide range of outpatient services to complement its traditional core of inpatient services. Whereas most hospitals were freestanding, independent institutions in 1975, a growing number now belong to hospital systems or networks. Some hospitals have also vertically integrated by buying physician practices and developing their own insurance products.

The environment in which hospitals operate has changed as well. Hospitals face a new and important class of purchasers. Concurrently, there have been major changes in how they are reimbursed. In 1975, hospitals operated in an environment of "patient-driven competition," in which shopping decisions were relegated to patients and their physicians. Reimbursement was typically based on a hospital's average cost of providing services. Today, hospitals operate in an environment of "payer-driven" competition, in which the locus of control over decisions about what care to buy and where to buy it has increasingly shifted toward payers—managed-care plans, employers, and government agencies (Dranove, Shanley, and White 1993). At the same time, traditional, cost-based reimbursement has largely disappeared. Private insurers typically negotiate prices with hospitals on an individual basis, while Medicare sets prices administratively on a prospective basis independent of individual hospitals' costs.

In this study, we consider the evolving structure of the hospital industry since 1975. The forces driving recent shifts in the industry have been complex. On the demand side, both political and economic forces have played an important role in determining volume and structure. On the supply side, technological and organizational forces have had a major impact not only on the types of services available and on their costs, but also on the costs of obtaining information about clinical and financial performance.

To sort out the interactions among these various forces, we draw on two key insights from the literature on health economics:

• The evolution of healthcare institutions reflects uncertainty about demand and difficulties in evaluating the appropriateness and quality of care.

• There are economies of scope and scale in the production of many healthcare services, and these economies affect the desirability of horizontal and vertical integration.[1]

These insights provide a powerful framework for examining the structure of the healthcare industry as it existed in the 1970s and its subsequent evolution. We organize our analysis around two central questions. First, how have responses by the hospital industry to the changing healthcare environment been shaped by informational issues? Second, what has been the role of technology in this process?

In our analysis, we make no attempt to survey fully the vast literature on the hospital industry that has emerged since 1975. Rather, our goal is to present "stylized facts" useful in thinking about major trends. We seek to direct interested readers toward appropriate sources for more in-depth analyses, but we make no claims to be comprehensive.

Chapter 2 describes some of the central institutional features of the healthcare industry, explores how problems with information shape these institutions, and examines ways in which technology may affect the choice of institutional arrangements. Chapter 3 considers the hospital industry in the era of patient-driven competition, circa 1975. Chapter 4 examines trends since 1975 and the shift from patient-driven to payer-driven competition. Chapter 5 considers the hospital industry at the end of the 1990s. Chapter 6 explores the implications of the recent experiences.

Before proceeding, a brief discussion of terminology is appropriate. In this analysis, we focus on community hospitals. These are general hospitals, including teaching hospitals, that render a full complement of short-term, acute-care services to the community at large. These hospitals form the core of the U.S. hospital industry. But hospital care is also provided in a variety of other settings. That includes hospitals rendering care to defined populations—for example, military service veterans, prisoners, or students. Care also includes specialty hospitals, particularly psychiatric hospitals, and specialized units with inpatient beds, such as drug treatment facilities. In 1996 an estimated 82 percent of hospital spending went toward community hospital services; the remaining 18 percent went toward other forms of hospital care (American Hospital Association 1998; National Center for Health Statistics 1998). Wherever possible, statistics reported in this study refer to community hospitals. In some cases, however, data are available only for hospitals as a group and are reported as such.

2

Uncertainty, Technology, and the Organization of Hospitals

T he healthcare industry has a number of distinctive institutional features that have persisted over time:

- Patients pay directly for only a fraction of the cost of care. Especially in the case of hospital care, most of the cost is covered by insurance.
- Patients depend on physicians to act as agents in their behalf. Physicians provide services and oversee the delivery of care.
- Nonprofit organizations dominate many segments of healthcare delivery, and particularly hospital care.

We believe that these institutional arrangements did not arise by accident. Rather, they represent reasonable responses to problems that patients face in the healthcare marketplace. As the nature of these problems changes, whether because of internal tensions or changes in the market environment, the institutional arrangements may be expected to evolve. We shall explore how that might happen.

Uncertain Demand and Insurance

The demand for most consumer goods and services is relatively predictable. In contrast, it is frequently difficult for consumers to predict when they will fall ill. Moreover, care may be very costly in the event of illness. Insurance enables consumers to protect themselves against these unpredictable financial risks. But insurance comes at a price. First there are the administrative costs associated with marketing, tracking claims, and underwriting. In addition, generously insured patients may use costly services that provide little or no benefit in terms of improved outcomes. (Economists call this moral hazard.) Generously insured consumers also have little incentive to comparison-shop among providers to obtain the lowest price. Thus, providers may raise their prices, further driving up medical costs.

Insurers may attempt to limit these problems by requiring patients to make copayments, but their ability to impose copayments is limited. Patients object to meaningful copayments because these would increase their exposure to financial risk—the vulnerability against which they purchased insurance in the first place. Insurers may instead or additionally limit consumer choice of services and providers, and direct consumers to those providers who offer the lowest prices and the least costly mix of services. But under this strategy, at the heart of what has become known as *managed care*, patients run the risk of receiving inadequate or inappropriate care. This is especially problematic when patients are unable to determine for themselves whether they are receiving the right care.

Imperfect Information and the Choice of Care

Most healthcare consumers lack the information and expertise to determine confidently what services they should purchase. Likewise, it is often difficult for them to evaluate whom they should purchase services from. There are many reasons for this.

In most markets, consumers learn about quality through repeated use of the product. Fortunately, most of us are infrequent users of healthcare services. In fact, we may purchase specific services, such as maternity care or a total hip replacement, only once or twice. Sometimes we purchase services repeatedly—for example, asthmatics purchase hospital services for severe attacks. On other occasions, we may draw on the accumulated experiences of friends and relatives who have had similar medical needs. Even then, the complex and idiosyncratic nature of medicine makes it difficult for consumers to develop sufficient knowledge and expertise to judge what services they need or evaluate the quality of providers. Consumers need both basic medical knowledge and idiosyncratic knowledge, along with the ability to assess their own symptoms.

The Use of Agents to Coordinate Care

In response to these problems, patients rely on physicians to make medical decisions on their behalf. Acting as agents for their patients, physicians use their specialized knowledge and skill, built upon years of education and experience, to diagnose ailments, recommend treatments, and coordinate the delivery of these treatments. Thus, they not only recommend and deliver treatments themselves but oversee the care of their patients in hospitals. In short, patients rely on physicians to act as captains of the ship in navigating them through the healthcare system. Patients trust their physician-agents to make wise choices, and their trust is enhanced by professional standards that discourage physicians from exploiting their superior knowledge for personal gain (Mechanic 1998).

The use of physician-agents poses its own problems, however. The Hippocratic Oath cannot eliminate self-interest. Physician-agents may abuse their trust. They may, for example, overprovide or underprovide services, provide care of substandard quality, or sacrifice patients' interests for their own convenience. Where such abuses are readily detected, they do not constitute a major problem; patients may rely on the market (they take their business elsewhere) and the courts (through malpractice laws) to discipline physicians who perform poorly. But for the very reason that patients employ physician-agents in the first place—that is, limited information—patients are ill-equipped to evaluate agents' performances (Arrow 1963).

Physician agency poses another problem. Individually, patients would like their physicians to provide all services whose expected value equals or exceeds the out-of-pocket cost. Collectively, however, patients would like physicians to provide services whose expected value equals or exceeds the full cost, thereby eliminating the inefficiencies associated with moral hazard. In this context, a patient would almost prefer his or her physician to act in the interest of the insurer, rather than in his or her own individual interest.

The design of the agency relationship between physicians and patients must address these problems. A key insight of the economic theory of agency is that the structure of agency relationships may be sensitive to: (1) how consumers and their agents trade off the costs and benefits of different actions, and (2) information costs. Thus, healthcare consumers and policymakers must balance the cost and quality of care when deciding how to structure the agency relationship. One key aspect of the balance involves choices about how physicians should be paid—for example, between fee-for-service and capitation. (Traditionally, insurers paid physicians on a fee-for-service basis, so that the physician received additional payments for each service rendered. Increasingly, insurers pay physicians a fixed fee per patient, or capitation, that is independent of the level of services.) In addition, consumers must weigh the benefits of monitoring and evaluating physician-agents against the costs of gathering information. Here options include gathering more information themselves, hiring private third parties, or turning to public regulation—for example, occupational licensure laws.

Nonprofit Institutions

Although physicians act as coordinators of care, the majority of services are actually delivered by other providers. Most notable are institutional providers, especially hospitals. As noted, nonprofit organization of hospitals is common. Agency considerations may play a key role in this. Consumers may rely on nonprofit institutions for many of the same reasons they rely on physician-agents. Profit-seeking organizations may be tempted to exploit consumers by providing substandard levels of hard-to-measure attributes. A for-profit hospital, for example, might hire inadequately trained personnel at low wages. If consumers are unable to observe the quality of the personnel, they may continue to purchase services at that hospital, thereby enriching the hospital's owners. In nonprofit organizations, constraints on the distribution of profits may curtail these incentives. Hansmann (1980) and Weisbrod (1988, 1989) argue that nonprofits do not have the same temptation to shirk on quality, both because the owners have a genuine interest in serving the public interest and because, even if they did shirk, they could not be assured of the resulting profits. Patients intuitively understand this, and naturally seek out nonprofit providers.[2]

Nonprofits may dominate the hospital sector, but they are relatively unimportant in most other markets. One reason is that nonprofits have limited access to capital and may be slow to exploit new market opportunities. Another reason may be that nonprofits are inefficient. Lacking a clear metric for performance evaluation, substandard managers who might not survive in a for-profit firm can survive in a nonprofit organization. The theory of agency suggests that the prevalence of nonprofits may be sensitive to the ability of consumers (or their representatives) to measure quality, and to the trade-off between cost and quality. Accordingly, reductions in the costs of obtaining information on quality or greater willingness to trade off reduced costs for quality may lead to reduced reliance on nonprofits.

Technology

Technology may play an important role in the evolving structure of healthcare institutions in two ways—through changes in the technology of providing medical care and through changes in information technology. It is widely understood that over time, changes in medical technology have been a major determinant of the cost and quality of care (*see* Newhouse 1992, Weisbrod 1991). As Weisbrod (1991) observes, technology could either increase or decrease costs. On balance, however, technological change has been associated with increasing costs. New technologies, such as transplants, chemotherapy, prosthetic devices, and so forth, tend to increase the costs of treating particular diseases. Changes in the "intensity" of care associated with new technologies have been a major factor in the growth of healthcare costs, accounting for about a third of the total growth in healthcare spending between 1963 and 1996 (National Center for Health Statistics 1998).

Through its effects on cost and quality, technological change may affect the optimal structure of agency relationships. For example, the further introduction of cost-increasing technology might increase the attractiveness of capitation because of the incentives it gives providers to curtail utilization. Cost pressures may also increase the political attractiveness of a single-payer healthcare system, whose national budgeting process might place a lid on rising costs. Conversely, changes that boost quality may increase the attractiveness of fee-for-service payment, while reducing political pressures for systemic reforms.

Technology can also affect the structure of agency relationships by making available low-cost information that providers and consumers can use to evaluate the cost and quality of care. Providers may integrate to enable them to share valuable information that can be used to create practice guidelines. Health Maintenance Organizations and Preferred Provider Organizations may use quality and cost information to exclude certain providers from networks. Some observers have even suggested that consumers can use web-based information to directly monitor their physicians' choices (Herzlinger 1997; Milkenson 1997), thereby reducing their need to rely on physician-agents. Nevertheless, the sheer volume and complexity of healthcare information might increase the value of physicians or other agents who are able to make sense of the data.

3

The Hospital Industry in 1975: The Era of Patient-driven Competition

U p until the early 1980s, hospitals and the rest of the healthcare sector all operated in a market environment of patient-driven competition. Before looking in detail at the hospital industry circa 1975, we draw on the framework developed in chapter 2 to consider briefly some of the main features of this market environment and its implications for costs and quality.

Patient-driven Competition

Under patient-driven competition, patients and their doctors were responsible for shopping for care. Guided by their physician-agents, patients made decisions about what care to buy and from whom to buy it. The bulk of care was paid for by insurance, which took the form either of employer-sponsored private insurance or public-sponsored insurance under the Medicare and Medicaid programs. Except for a few Health Maintenance Organizations (HMOs), there was little integration between insurers and providers. Private insurers and public programs served simply as conduits for funds, validating patients' choices. Through the 1980s, most insurers paid physicians on a fee-for-service basis, while payments to hospitals were usually based on their average costs of care. Insurers reviewed claims to determine whether hospitals accurately listed the services rendered and correctly reported their costs. But they did not attempt to hold providers accountable for the appropriateness or cost of care. Under these arrangements, more care meant more money for doctors and hospitals. This gave physicians a financial interest to provide as many services as they could, and hospitals had no reason to object. At the same time, patient copayments were usually small, so patients had little reason to object either, as long as they perceived that the services would provide even a small benefit.

That arrangement had two important implications for providers. First, because insured patients were largely insulated from price, patients' decisions about which hospitals to use were likely to be made primarily on the basis of providers' perceived quality, amenities, and patient convenience rather than on the basis of price. Second, hospitals and other providers could expect to be reimbursed for whatever services these patients used. The combined incentives caused hospitals to focus on attracting insured patients to their facilities on the basis of nonprice characteristics, confident that they would recover the costs of treatments provided to those patients irrespective of their level of need.

In this context, Robinson and Luft (1985), Kopit and McCann (1988), and others raise the possibility that hospital competition may lead to a "medical arms race" (MAR), in which prices are higher in more competitive markets because of quality competition. Interestingly, however, Noether (1988), while finding evidence that there may be more quality competition in more competitive markets, finds no evidence that list prices in 1977–1978 are higher in more competitive markets.

At the systemic level, particularly in retrospect, patient-driven competition had obvious cost disadvantages. It is widely recognized that the combination of fee-for-service payment and generous cost-based insurance created three costly incentives. First, insurance created a classic "commons problem"—that is, a situation in which each individual's selfish behavior leaves all individuals worse off. As discussed, insurance may lead to moral hazard in consumption decisions. Patients demanded (and physicians and hospitals willingly provided) treatments of even marginal value. Second, insured patients had little incentive to shop around for the best prices, enabling providers to set prices in excess of marginal costs. Third, physicians who were paid on a fee-for-service basis had financial incentives to recommend and provide treatments of marginal value merely to enhance their own incomes. Economists call this "demand inducement."

It is important to recognize, however, that patient-driven competition had important attractions from the perspective of patients. Physicians, acting in their capacity as the agents of individual patients, helped their patient-principals to navigate an increasingly complex healthcare system. They could make sensible healthcare-purchasing decisions and could coordinate the myriad of resources needed for effective treatment. Patients had substantial choice of provider, although in reality they usually obtained services from the providers recommended to them by their primary care practitioner (PCP).[3] Physicians had financial incentives to err on the side of over-providing services, which may have enhanced quality. Physicians also faced little price competition, which may have encouraged them to compete more heavily on the basis of quality (Dranove and Satterthwaite 1992).

Any shift away from that system raised issues of cost-against-quality trade-offs. In examining subsequent events, however, it would be a mistake to view the cost implications of patient-driven competition as its only drawback. Cost aside, the use of individual physician-agents does not necessarily solve consumers' shopping problems. All physicians are not equally good agents. Some may lack the requisite technical knowledge, while others may be poor coordinators of care. However much a patient may want a quality agent, he or she would be hard pressed to identify the best physician-agents. In 1975 it was all but impossible for patients to gather systematic evidence on the efficacy of their physicians. Instead, they had to rely on intangibles such as bedside manner and reputation. Everyone wanted Marcus Welby, but no one had a systematic basis for evaluating whether he was a competent doctor.

Moreover, however much physicians may have wanted to be good coordinators of their patients' care, they would have found it hard to do so. There was no easy way for physicians to assess systematically the quality and costs of their peers and of institutions such as hospitals. Instead, they had to rely on their personal knowledge, word of mouth, and reputation. Physicians often developed referral networks based mainly on friendships and convenience. It was also difficult for physicians to keep abreast of the benefits and costs of new medical innovations. Physicians drew very different conclusions about the efficacy of specific interventions, leading to the well-known small-area variations in medical practice (*see* Phelps and Mooney 1993 for a review).

In 1975 there was virtually no framework, however imperfect, in place for payers to offer an alternative to evaluation of quality by individual patients and their doctors. When we turn to developments since the early 1980s and the shift from patient-driven to payer-driven competition in chapter 4, we explore an important secondary theme—changes in the potential ability of payers to assess quality.

The Industry in 1975

In 1975 there were 5,875 community general hospitals, with some 942,000 beds (see table 3–1). The average hos-

TABLE 3–1
COMMUNITY HOSPITAL CHARACTERISTICS, 1928–1996

Hospital Characteristics	1928	1946	1955	1965	1975	1985	1996
Number of community hospitals:							
Nonprofit	1,889	2,584	3,097	3,426	3,339	3,349	3,045
Government	540	785	1,120	1,453	1,761	1,578	1,330
Investor-owned	1,877	1,076	1,020	857	775	805	759
Total	4,306	4,445	5,237	5,736	5,875	5,732	5,134
Number of community hospital beds: (1000s)							
Nonprofit	197	301	389	515	658	707	598
Government	81	133	142	179	210	189	155
Investor-owned	58	39	37	47	73	104	109
Total	336	473	568	741	942	1,001	862
Average number of beds per hospital							
Nonprofit	104	117	126	150	197	211	196
Government	150	169	127	123	119	120	117
Investor-owned	31	36	36	55	95	129	144
All community hospitals	78	106	109	129	160	175	168

SOURCES: 1928–1965: William D. White, "The American Hospital Industry since 1900: A Short History," in R. Scheffler and L. Rossiter, eds., *Advances in Health Services Research*, vol. 3 (Greenwich Conn.: JAI Press 1982). 1975–1996: National Center for Health Statistics, *Health, United States 1998* DHHS Publication (PHS) 98-1232, 1998.

pital had 160 beds. While half of all hospitals were quite small (fewer than 100 beds), small hospitals accounted for only 16 percent of beds. Slightly more than half of all beds, 52 percent, were in medium-sized hospitals (100 to 399 beds), and the remaining 32 percent of beds were in large hospitals (399 beds or more). The average occupancy rate for hospitals was 75 percent, and the average length of stay was 7.7 days (American Hospital Association 1976).

Against a background of patient-driven competition, hospitals in 1975 shared a number of common charac- teristics:

- Community general hospitals were truly general, providing a wide range of inpatient services but relatively limited outpatient services.
- They served local markets.
- They were freestanding, locally controlled organizations with important links to their communities; horizontal integration was limited.
- Vertical integration was also limited. Hospital medical staffs were autonomous, and links to payer organizations were rare.
- Most hospitals were nonprofit.
- The bulk of hospital revenues came from private insurance and public programs.
- Purchasers rarely compared hospitals systematically on the basis of cost or quality.

Below we examine each of these features in turn. We argue that this bundle of common characteristics represented a reasonable and efficient response to problems with the delivery of acute medical services, given existing economies of scale and scope and agency issues.

Range of Services

Inpatient services formed the core business of virtually all hospitals. Following a pattern established at the beginning of the century, hospitals of all sizes centralized the production of a broad selection of inpatient services under one roof (White 1990). Thus, the typical community hospital provided maternity care, major surgical procedures, and treatment of complex medical problems like chronic obstructive pulmonary disease and cardiovascular disease.

Hospital involvement in outpatient care was more limited. As of 1975, outpatient services accounted for only 11.9 percent of total hospital revenues. Hospital-based home healthcare and skilled nursing care were virtually nonexistent. Even organized outpatient departments were uncommon; remarkably, in 1975 only 26 percent of community hospitals reported they had outpatient departments (American Hospital Association 1976).

Economies of scope offer a powerful explanation for why hospitals offered a wide range of inpatient services. The production of hospital services involves a number of inputs that can be applied to the treatment of many diseases. These include nursing services, diagnostic facilities, intensive care units, surgical suites, and pharmacy services. Economies arise as hospitals spread the fixed costs of these inputs across more units of output, or as they more fully utilize excess staff and equipment that are required to meet volatile demand (Cowing et al. 1983; Lynk 1995). Hospitals could, in principle, achieve these economies by producing large numbers of a handful of treatments. Thus, one could imagine highly specialized hospitals each rendering a particular type of treatment (such as cancer care or cardiovascular care), assuming sufficient demand in a hospital's market area to enable it to fully exploit potential economies.

Economies of scope extend beyond production. Hospitals may enjoy reputational economies of scope. Such economies have clearly benefited the nationally renowned Mayo Clinic and Cleveland Clinic, which have opened facilities around the nation. They may also benefit local hospitals with strong reputations. In addition, it may be easier to coordinate outpatient and inpatient activities (such as medical recordkeeping) if the facilities have a common owner.

Economies of scope not only help explain the existence of the general hospital, they also explain the existence of two broad types of general hospitals: those providing primary and secondary services, and those providing tertiary services. Hospitals in the first group offer basic services and may perform relatively unsophisticated procedures, such as appendectomies and normal vaginal deliveries, and they treat patients when there is not a demand for complex services. Tertiary-care hospitals provide those "simple" treatments, but they also provide complex treatments such as neonatal intensive care, organ transplants, and megavoltage radiation treatment of cancer patients.

Economies of scale explain why relatively few hospitals provided complex treatments. But economies of scope explain why the same hospital that provided one complex treatment tended to provide others. Tertiary-care hospitals acquired the staffing and equipment necessary to provide relatively rare treatments for severely ill patients. They exploited economies of scope by spreading their specialized skills across a range of treatments. Even in dense urban areas capable of supporting many hospitals, general hospitals, as opposed to hospitals specializing in a few clinical areas, were the norm.[4]

It is difficult to measure the magnitude of scope economies. Athey and Stern (1998) review the methodological literature on economies of scope and offer a number of techniques for assessing them. They suggest that a good starting point is to observe whether services are offered in tandem. We see ample evidence of that for hospitals. For example, virtually all hospitals treat the same core set of twenty to thirty Diagnosis Related Groups

(DRGs) that typically account for 50 percent of all hospital admissions. To take another example, hospitals that have offered specialized diagnostic services, such as computerized tomographic (CT) scans, have also tended to offer specialized surgical services, such as coronary artery bypass graft surgery (CABG). (Some hospitals offer CT scans but not CABG surgery, but seldom does a hospital offer CABG but not CT scans.) Hospitals specializing in a particular disease, however, are rare.

Athey and Stern (1998) note that these patterns are consistent with scope economies but could also reflect economies of scale at the level of individual services, managerial complementarities, or the effect of some omitted factor that leads to particular patterns of service offerings. They suggest a number of complex statistical techniques to sort through these competing explanations. But the data needed to pass an Athey-Stern test of scope economies are unavailable (one would need identifiers that shift the cost of providing some but not other services, as well as measures of service productivity). Hence, while it is reasonable to conclude from existing data (and very reasonable to conclude from economic theory) that there are economies of scope, conclusive evidence is lacking.

Hospitals that fail to treat a wide range of diseases stand to miss out on more than just economies of scope. It is unlikely that physicians would admit their patients to hospitals that specialized narrowly in a handful of treatments. At the time of hospitalization, physicians may be uncertain about their patients' precise medical needs. They may therefore prefer to admit their patients to a hospital that is capable of treating a range of conditions. That is especially true if it would be costly to transfer the patient to another hospital once the diagnosis was made. Thus, patients, through their physician-agents, may have option-demand for a hospital that can treat a wide range of illnesses (Dranove and White 1996).

Although hospitals may not specialize their service offerings, they may specialize in the populations they serve (Dranove, White, and Wu 1993). The most obvious examples are county hospitals, which treat a disproportionate percentage of low-income patients who are enrolled in public insurance programs or who lack insurance altogether. Some hospitals have strong links to religious groups. As we discuss below, many hospitals draw patients largely from their local communities, leading to further segmentation based on demographic factors. Economies of scope and option-demand also explain why hospitals may provide inpatient and outpatient care at a single facility.[5] Many of the inputs necessary to produce inpatient care, including diagnostic, pharmacy, and laboratory services, can be used to produce outpatient care. At the same time, patients seeking certain outpatient services, such as surgery, may prefer to receive them at a hospital-based outpatient facility. That way, sophisticated inpatient services would be readily available in the event that something should go wrong.

But patients may prefer to purchase certain outpatient services from providers other than hospitals. Non-hospital providers of outpatient services (for example, a doctor in his or her office) generally offer greater convenience, ambience, and amenities. Non-hospital providers also generally offer lower prices for similar services. That may seem surprising, inasmuch as hospitals benefit from scope economies. But hospitals often have higher labor costs. Moreover, hospitals have tended to base their prices on average costs rather than incremental costs (Goldsmith 1980). Burdened with the high overhead associated with inpatient care, those hospitals that based their prices for outpatient care on average costs have set higher prices than have dedicated outpatient providers. It is important to note that the price differential has not necessarily reflected differences in the incremental cost of care.

We can infer from the limited involvement of hospitals in outpatient services in 1975 that those concerns predominated. At the same time, the potential for hospitals to reap economies of scope from outpatient services had important implications for the years to follow.

Geographic Markets

In 1975, hospitals sold their services locally (McGuirk and Porell 1984). A typical "big city" hospital drew 80 percent or more of its patients from its local metropolitan area. An exception was major tertiary-care hospitals, especially those in mid-sized markets that were referral centers for surrounding communities. Most residents of large cities turned to their local hospitals for services, but residents of smaller communities frequently traveled to urban areas, particularly for complex and difficult treatments (Morrisey, Sloan, and Valvona 1988).

Hospital services were local for several reasons. One obvious reason is that travel is costly. Not only must a patient travel to and from the hospital; friends and relatives may have to make several trips for visitation. That raises the cost of going outside the local community for care. In addition, with generous insurance, as discussed above, there was little incentive for patients to shop on the basis of price. Hence, a lower price alone was unlikely to attract patients to a distant hospital.

Quality could, of course, still be an important motive for travel. But that raises other important reasons for relying on local providers, based on agency theory. Patients relied on primary-care physicians and their referral networks to select a hospital for inpatient care. Physicians usually preferred local hospitals, both for convenience and concerns about quality—physicians will generally provide better care if they work with the same medical staff on a repeated basis. Physicians also had extensive personal knowledge of local hospitals and could readily identify a local hospital that had the desired services and quality. In addition, patients themselves have been more familiar with the reputations of local hospitals, and may have been reluctant to go to a hospital that they know nothing about, unless local hospitals do not offer the desired service. Exceptions such as the Mayo Clinic and the Cleveland Clinic, which attracted patients nationwide, may have proven the rule; they were among a small handful of provider groups in the United States with national reputations.

Community Links, Horizontal Integration, and Local Control

Most hospitals were started by local organizations such as churches, universities, and community groups. Over time, they established local brand names and became among the most trusted institutions in their communities. The majority were centerpieces for local fund-raising activities, and business leaders vied for membership on nonprofit hospital boards. Local brand reputations remained strong through 1975, and community hospitals retained local control. Ermann and Gabel (1984) estimate that, in 1975, 75 percent of all community hospitals were independent, freestanding institutions, including the vast majority of urban hospitals.

The importance of local reputation helps to explain why so few urban hospitals belonged to national systems. The need for a local reputation did not preclude the formation of local systems, however. The predominance of freestanding hospitals suggests either that economies of scale and scope across hospitals were minimal, or that patient-driven competition did not create incentives to attempt to realize such economies.

Autonomous Medical Staffs and Vertical Integration

Another striking feature of virtually all hospitals in 1975 was the absence of vertical integration. Although accepted as captains of the ship, most physicians did not work for the ship owners. Instead, physicians were independent business men and women to whom the hospitals granted substantial decisionmaking authority about treatment decisions. Thus, physicians were captains of the team in hospitals, and they directed hospital staffs in clinical matters (Fuchs 1983). But they usually billed independently for their services, while hospital medical staffs were typically autonomous and subject to minimal controls by hospitals (Stevens 1989). At the same time that physicians remained independent of hospitals, hospitals maintained their independence from other parts of the vertical chain. Few offered insurance or were owned by payer organizations. Nor was involvement in freestanding outpatient facilities or in nursing homes common.

A few HMOs did vertically integrate. Some staff- and group-model HMOs, including Kaiser and the Group Health Cooperative (GHC), simultaneously offered insurance and owned their own hospitals. GHC employed its physicians, while Kaiser contracted with large physician groups (the Permanente groups) whose members worked exclusively for the HMO at a fixed salary. But in 1975, only a tiny fraction of physicians was involved.

Agency problems help to explain the autonomy of physicians. If physicians have an ownership stake in the hospital, or even if their compensation is directly based on the financial well-being of their hospital, then they might have even greater incentive to induce demand for costly inpatient services. Patients might therefore prefer independent physicians, particularly if they are at for-profit hospitals (White 1982). In addition, autonomous physicians have a free hand to take the patient's side when coordinating care in a complex hospital environment. Administrators in both nonprofit and for-profit hospitals might be too bound by bureaucracy to ensure adequately that patients' idiosyncratic needs are met (Harris 1977). Consistent with that circumstance, conflicts with hospitals over physician autonomy have historically been most intense for hospital-based specialists such as pathologists and radiologists, who provide technical services and usually do not act as patients' agents (Stevens 1971).

Two additional factors may help to explain the dominance of physician autonomy. First, physicians (like many other professionals) may value independence for its own sake. Second, it may have been difficult for hospitals (especially nonprofits) to pay competitive salaries to physicians (White 1979).

Investor-owned versus Nonprofit Organization

Only 13 percent of hospitals in 1975 were for-profits, and they accounted for only 8 percent of total beds (National Center for Health Statistics 1998). For-profit hospitals shared many features with nonprofit and government hospitals. They competed in local markets, produced a wide variety of services, and in most cases had autonomous medical staffs.[6] There were three important differences between for-profits and other hospitals. First, for-profits were typically small; their average size was ninety-five beds (National Center for Health Statistics 1998). Second, they were disproportionately located in smaller towns, where they were often the only hospitals. And third, by 1975, for-profit hospitals were joining national systems such as the Hospital Corporation of America and Humana, whereas nonprofits remained independent.

Two factors are important in explaining why most hospitals were nonprofits. First, nonprofit hospitals have historically been the "vendors of last resort" and dispensers of charity care. As discussed by Weisbrod (1988, 1989), communities showed altruistic concern by providing tax breaks and contributions to nonprofits for charity care. Unable to monitor directly how the funds were used, communities may have been reluctant to do the same with for-profit hospitals. As Weisbrod observes, an alternative would have been simply to buy care with charitable funds from for-profit institutions. But in any case, as discussed below, most nonprofit hospitals provided relatively little outright charity care.

A second and probably more important factor is that nonprofit hospitals were attractive to patients who were concerned about the quality and appropriateness of care but were unable to determine readily which hospitals were the best. On the one hand, these patients may have worried that investor-owned hospitals would take advantage of their ignorance about quality. On the other hand, they might have believed that nonprofit hospitals would provide higher quality, particularly on those dimensions of quality that are hard to evaluate (Weisbrod 1988, 1989). In that way, nonprofit organizations may have reduced the shopping problems faced by uninformed healthcare consumers. It is interesting to note that in the early part of the twentieth century, many hospitals were initially for-profit ventures established by physicians as extensions of their medical practices. There was a rapid shift toward the nonprofit format, however, as community support for hospitals grew (Marmor, Schlesinger, and Smithey 1986; White 1982).

Theorists have identified a number of potentially important differences between nonprofit and for-profit hospitals, but the evidence is inconclusive. For-profits tend to have higher prices and to provide less uncompensated care. Both of those differences may be attributable more to location than to managerial objectives, although location itself may be endogenous (Norton and Staiger 1994). Researchers have yet to provide compelling evidence of differences in quality. Sloan et al. (1998), for example, find that nonprofits have 2 percent lower inpatient mortality rates, but their empirical methods lack statistical power, and the difference is not statistically significant. Lastly, Lynk (1996) found that nonprofits do not exploit market power in a manner consistent with traditional theories of competition, which suggests a relaxation of antitrust enforcement. Subsequent research by Dranove and Ludwick (1999) and Keeler, Melnick, and Zwanziger (1999), however, contradicts Lynk's findings.

Hospital Revenue Sources

Table 3–2 reports data on revenue sources for hospitals, including noncommunity hospitals. In 1975 patients paid directly (out of pocket) for only 8 percent of hospital services. Private insurance paid for a third, while the public sector (mainly Medicare, Medicaid, and local taxes going to county hospitals) paid for 56 percent. Private charity paid for no more than 3 percent of hospital expenses.

These figures suggest that the public sector provided the bulk of charity care. But that conclusion is clouded by the potential for cross-subsidies. Hospitals could use profits from privately insured patients to subsidize care for the indigent. Of course, if hospitals were unable to extract profits from paying patients, they would be forced to reduce such subsidies (Morrisey 1994), a point we will re-

TABLE 3–2
Sources of Hospital Revenues, All Hospital Care, 1965–1996

	1965	1970	1975	1980	1985	1990	1996
Total expenditures (billions)	14.0	28.0	52.6	102.7	168.3	256.4	358.5
Percent distribution:							
Out-of-pocket payments	19.6	9.0	8.3	5.2	5.2	4.0	2.6
Private health insurance	40.9	32.4	32.9	35.5	35.0	36.9	31.6
Other private funds	1.9	3.2	2.7	4.9	4.9	4.2	4.3
Government:							
Medicaid	—	9.5	10.0	10.3	9.3	11.5	14.7
Medicare	—	19.2	22.0	25.7	29.1	27.3	33.0
Total federal, state, and local government	37.6	55.4	56.0	54.4	54.8	56.6	61.5

SOURCE: National Center for Health Statistics, *Health, United States 1998* DHHS Publication (PHS) 98-1232, 1998.

visit below in the context of the growth of managed care and increasing price competition.

Quality and Cost Data

Hospitals in 1975 were accredited by the Joint Commission on Hospital Accreditation (JCHA), now the Joint Commission on Accreditation of Healthcare Organizations (JCAHO). JCHA accreditation was based largely on structural features (such as staffing and equipment requirements) rather than on outcomes. Yet there was no systematic source of data that would enable consumers to compare the clinical performance of hospitals. Consumers also found it difficult to obtain price information. Hospitals posted their charges for selected services (like a day in the medical/surgical ward), but did not post prices for treatments. They often bundled services very differently, so that a hospital with a low price per service might have a high price per treatment. That made comparison shopping for the best price all but impossible.

Access to quality and price information was limited both by the available technology and by institutional factors. Large-scale computer databases were not available. Collecting and analyzing data involved high levels of skill and substantial cost. Standard formats for collecting data were also lacking. Finally, many physicians resisted efforts to promote data collection, justly apprehending that that would enable hospitals and insurers to intervene in the doctor-patient relationship.

4
The Evolving Hospital Marketplace

U p until the mid-1970s, patient-driven competition was tolerated despite the issues we have discussed regarding costs and quality. By the late 1970s, two types of factors created growing pressure for change. First, public policy (Medicare and Medicaid), demographic shifts, and new technology all contributed to rapid increases in medical expenditures.[7] Second, a revolution was taking place in healthcare management information systems. Improvements in healthcare data systems not only aided internal management decisionmaking but also provided cost and quality data with which payers could systematically compare providers. These data systems also allowed payers to develop and implement more complex forms of reimbursement. We discuss each of these factors in more detail below.

Pressure for Change

During the 1966–1975 period, healthcare costs (adjusted for inflation) grew by an average of 6.5 percent annually. Between 1965 and 1975, as shown in table 1–1, the share of national income spent on healthcare rose from 5.7 percent to 8 percent. By 1980, it had reached 8.9 percent, a more-than-50 percent increase from 1965 (National Center for Health Statistics 1998). Persistent increases in costs led a growing number of policymakers and students of healthcare to question whether the benefits of unfettered physician agency were worth the costs.

Also during this period, major advances were made in information technology. With the development of high-speed computer systems it became possible to create centralized, large-scale databases that could be used to gather and analyze financial and clinical information. (The best known and most frequently used is the MEDPAR Medicare claims database.) These systems have obvious applications for internal administrative purposes—for example, cost-accounting and billing. As discussed below, they opened the way for the creation of standardized data sets that were designed for regulatory purposes but that offered a range of possible applications for external evaluation of financial and clinical performance.

It is relatively straightforward to describe the changes associated with the emergence of payer-driven competition. It is more difficult, and beyond the scope of this study, to explain why payer-driven competition emerged when other industrial nations adopted more centralized, budget-driven approaches (*see* Arnould, Rich, and White 1993). The emergence of a market-oriented cost-containment strategy was not a foregone conclusion. Rather, it grew out of a period of regulatory experimentation and intense political debate over the extent to which public policy should ensure access to care. As late as the Carter administration, comprehensive national health insurance was widely discussed. It reemerged as an issue in the Clinton administration in 1994, and it remains a continuing, if muted, concern. If a national health insurance scheme had been adopted, industry organization would probably look quite different. We take reliance on a market-driven system as a given in the analysis of industry development that follows, but we recognize that healthcare reform could potentially reemerge as an issue in the future.

The Changes Begin

Interestingly, despite the apparent dominance of market-based approaches to cost containment, Medicare and Medicaid were the first major payers systematically to address rising costs. Rather than directly attacking the agency problems that were the root cause of inefficiencies in the system, regulators focused on hospital services as the single most important component of the healthcare bill. Most states introduced "certificate of need" (CON) controls that limited hospital expansion, and CON was formalized as a standard by the federal government through the National Health Planning and Resources Development Act of 1974. A number of states also introduced hospital rate-setting programs that rewarded hospitals financially for reducing costs. That practice was formalized nationwide when the federal government's Health Care Finance Administration (HCFA) established its Prospective Payment System (PPS) for Medicare inpatient services, which was introduced for hospitals in 1983 (Smith 1992).

These regulatory actions had several important implications. First, the introduction of the PPS restructured incentives for hospitals and drove a wedge between doctors and hospitals. Second, government controls generated an increasingly complex regulatory environment for hospitals that created a demand for growing administrative sophistication. Third, PPS formulas included adjustments that favored certain types of hospitals, particularly large urban teaching hospitals.

Under the PPS, hospitals were placed at financial risk for the cost of inpatient services to a major source of admissions—Medicare enrollees, who accounted for nearly 30 percent of hospital expenditures in 1983 (National Center for Health Statistics 1988). Inpatients were classified on the basis of Diagnosis Related Group (DRG). With some important adjustments, discussed below, hospitals were reimbursed a flat amount per admission, determined prospectively on the basis of the costs of providing care to patients in a nationwide DRG.

The Medicare PPS introduced what Shleifer (1985) subsequently dubbed "yardstick competition" to hospital markets. As such, it was identified as a "pro-competitive" reform, even though it basically involved an administrative pricing scheme (Smith 1992). Under the PPS, the Medicare per admission payment for an episode of inpatient treatment was the yardstick against which each hospital's financial success was measured. Hospitals whose costs were lower than the DRG payment could keep any profit. But hospitals whose costs exceeded the DRG payment were at risk for any loss. As a result, incentives were created for hospitals to control services per inpatient admission.[8] Hospitals responded by reducing lengths of stay, laying off staff, shifting care to outpatient settings, and pursuing a variety of other cost-containment strategies (ProPAC 1997). For example, many hospitals adopted continuous quality-improvement programs; by 1992 the majority had done so.

Physicians continued to be paid on a traditional fee-for-service basis.[9] As in the past, the more services they provided, the more they were paid. Since, as patients' agents, physicians continued to oversee the coordination of care and to play a key role in determining the provision of inpatient services, obvious tensions arose. The interests of hospitals and doctors were no longer aligned with respect to inpatient services. There were, hence, clear incentives for hospitals to impose controls on their medical staffs with respect to these services, although traditional incentives remained in place for outpatient services.

It is important to emphasize, however, that despite innovations in payment incentives under the PPS and other regulatory programs, existing agency relationships between patients and physicians were largely untouched by public initiatives to control costs in the 1970s and early 1980s. The PPS created new tensions between doctors and hospitals that have subsequently been greatly amplified under managed care. But even in the case of the PPS, patients and their physicians remained firmly in control of shopping decisions about which care to buy and from whom to buy it. Indeed, even in 1999, Medicare remains perhaps the last major bastion of traditional, patient-driven competition in this respect.

Growing regulatory complexity also placed increased demands on hospital administrators. For example, certificate of need laws and planning requirements required hospitals to generate extensive reports to justify capital investments. Medicare and state rate-review systems imposed growing data collection requirements. The Medicare PPS required that hospitals classify patients by DRG and that they report data on utilization, and these requirements introduced standardized product lines for inpatient care (Smith 1992). HCFA also required hospitals to report department-level costs using a common cost-accounting methodology.

Data resulting from these requirements have been a major driver of private-sector change. HCFA made its clinical and cost data available to the public. Several states required their hospitals to report similar data. Some states, such as California, required hospitals to complete elaborate surveys of cost and utilization. Insurers and consulting firms would eventually use these data to compare hospitals on the basis of outcomes and costs, thereby catalyzing payer-driven competition.

A final aspect of public payment systems was to direct resources to particular types of hospitals. Three major types of payments have been involved: (1) Graduate Medical Education (GME) payments, based on hospitals' involvement in the graduate medical education of interns and residents; (2) Disproportionate Share Hospital (DSH) payments, to hospitals with high shares of low-income patients; (3) Medicare PPS Outlier payments, for unusually costly patients. The combined thrust of these payments has been to provide additional support for large, urban hospitals, particularly teaching institutions, many of which serve a social "safety net" function for the poor.

Medicare GME payments date from 1965, when the program was introduced. Currently, they take two forms: (1) Direct Medicare GME payments, based on the number of full-time-equivalent residents, and (2) Indirect Medical Education (IME) payments under the Medicare PPS, based on the ratio of interns and residents to beds in hospitals. In 1996, direct GME payments were $2.4 billion, IME payments were $4.3 billion, and hospitals received approximately an additional $1 billion for medical education under state Medicaid programs. Medical education payments not only support medical education; they also have important implications for the care of the poor in two ways. First, teaching hospitals tend to be located in large urban areas and to provide access to care for low-income populations concentrated in these areas. Second, to the extent that payments exceed costs, they may potentially be used to subsidize care for the poor at teaching hospitals (Fishman and Bentley 1997).

Disproportionate Share Hospital payments directly support hospitals with high proportions of low-income patients. Medicare DSH payments are based on hospital involvement in the care of Medicaid and Supplemental Security Income (SSI) patients. Medicaid DSH payments variously reflect hospitals' involvement in care for Medicaid and other low-income patients. DSH payments were introduced in 1981 for Medicaid and in 1986 for Medicare. They grew rapidly in the late 1980s, especially those for Medicaid, as a result of controversial manipulations of the program by states. Since the early 1990s, though, they have been relatively stable, following new legislation. In 1996,

Medicaid DSH payments came to about $19 billion, 12 percent of total program funding, and Medicare DSH payments were about $4.3 billion (Fishman and Bentley 1997).

Medicare Outlier payments were established in 1983, when the PPS was introduced. In 1997 they came to about $3 billion. Although all PPS hospitals are implicitly eligible for outlier payments, effectively the payments subsidize teaching hospitals and large urban safety net hospitals, because very high cost patients tend to be concentrated in these institutions (ProPAC 1997).

PPS operating payments for Outliers, IME, and DSH reflect the flow of these types of payments to particular groups of hospitals. In 1997, their combined total was about $12.2 billion, 17 percent of total PPS operating payments to hospitals for services. Of this $12.2 billion in Outlier, IME, and DHS payments, 43 percent went to major teaching hospitals, virtually all in urban areas. Large urban hospitals as a group received nearly 64 percent of these payments. For teaching hospitals, combined Outlier, IME, and DSH payments accounted for 37 percent of total Medicare revenue; for large urban hospitals, the combined share was more than 20 percent (ProPAC 1997). That distribution of funds has enabled large urban hospitals, particularly those engaged in teaching, to fare considerably better under the PPS than they would have fared otherwise. Medicaid DSH payments have further bolstered these hospitals.

The Private Sector Weighs In

In contrast with the public sector, private payers adopted a passive stance until the 1980s (Havighurst 1988). When finally galvanized into action, however, they introduced a series of changes in payment that fundamentally restructured agency relationships and, collectively, led to what has become known as *managed care*. The effect of those efforts has been to shift the locus of decisionmaking about what services to buy and from whom to buy them, away from patients and their physicians, to payers. That makes payers "super agents," both limiting and assisting the shopping decisions of patients and their physicians, and restructuring incentives for physicians to place them in a dual role—that is, agents of individual consumers but also, implicitly or explicitly, agents of payers.

The institutional origins of managed care date back more than half a century to prepaid group practices, including the predecessors to the Kaiser-Permanente Health Plans and the Group Health Cooperative (GHC) of Puget Sound. These tightly integrated organizations, which would eventually become known as Health Maintenance Organizations (HMOs), utilized exclusive panels of physicians and limited patient access to costly hospital services. By judiciously selecting physicians and monitoring their practice styles, these HMOs sought to eliminate many of the inefficiencies of the traditional system.

In the face of mounting pressure to control expenses, many health insurers in the 1980s sought to emulate key aspects of the Kaiser and GHC models. The most critical aspect was selectivity, which they implemented with the blessings of those who determined public policy. Until the early 1980s, state insurance-enabling laws effectively required most insurers to treat all providers equally. As a result, insurers had to reimburse for the services of a given provider, even if another provider in the same market offered the same services for a much lower price. Beginning in California in 1982, however, states started to drop these provisions. At the same time, many employers self-insured, thereby gaining exemption from state insurance regulation under the provisions of the Employee Retirement Income Security Act (ERISA) of 1974.

That allowed insurers and employers to contract selectively, on an arms-length basis, with a subset of physicians and hospitals, and to use financial incentives to steer patients toward these providers. With those changes, HMOs began to develop new institutional forms, such as network HMOs and Independent Practice Associations (IPAs). Other forms of Managed Care Organizations (MCOs) also began to appear, in particular Preferred Provider Organizations (PPOs), which selectively contracted on a fee-for-service basis. More recently, hybrid organizations such as Point of Service organizations (POSs) have taken market share from HMOs and PPOs. By 1995, more than 150 million Americans were enrolled in MCOs, while some 80 percent of all physicians had at least one MCO contract (Emmons and Simon 1996).

Selective contracting offered two benefits to insurers. First, by playing providers off against one another, insurers could obtain better prices than could their price-insensitive enrollees. Second, insurers could exclude providers whom they believed utilized resources inefficiently, had poor quality, or refused to participate in novel payment schemes. In practice, however, many MCOs merely refused to contract with providers who had high prices. But the ability of MCOs to negotiate lower prices was constrained by patient preferences. To be attractive to employers and their employees, MCOs' hospital networks must offer broad geographic coverage with few onerous access restrictions. Networks typically include at least half of all the hospitals in the local market, and it is not unusual for networks to include as many as 90 percent of local hospitals.[10] The consumer's desire for access may dilute MCO bargaining power. Consistent with that, evidence suggests that MCOs secure larger discounts when they are more exclusive (Town and Vistnes 1997).

The effect of selective contracting was to move healthcare markets toward the textbook model of perfect competition. A fundamental requirement of competitive markets is that purchasers are motivated to seek the best value and are able to identify the sellers who offer it. Through selective contracting, motivated and capable insurers shopped for medical services on behalf of unmotivated and less capable patients and physicians. In this way, selective contracting created the potential for a more competitive market for physician and hospital services.

In contrast with insured patients, who gained little if anything from lower costs, insurers were motivated to shop for the best value because they stood to gain from any cost savings. By lowering costs, they could realize increased profits and a potential competitive advantage in the market for health plans. In comparison with consumers, insurers were also potentially more capable shoppers, better able to realize economies of scale by efficiently gathering and analyzing price, utilization, and outcome data. A thriving support industry has emerged to provide independent assessments of the same data.[11]

Managed care has undeniably brought active competition to the healthcare marketplace. A large body of evidence shows that managed care has changed the demand for services. An equally large body of evidence shows that competition has driven down hospital prices, independent of the level of demand. (For reviews of this literature, *see* Dranove and White 1994 and Dranove and Satterthwaite forthcoming.)

There is considerable controversy at this time, however, about whether MCOs have focused on price at the possible expense of quality. The interests of MCOs are not necessarily aligned with those of consumers. Consumers or those acting on their behalf may, of course, impose market discipline on MCOs by shopping for plans. But that would presume that appropriate information is available to evaluate plan performance. It would also presume that employers, who make most plan selection decisions, fully account for the preferences of their employees. If either assumption were violated, consumer welfare might suffer.

5

The Hospital Industry in the Late 1990s: The Era of Payer-driven Competition

Evolving technology and the shift to payer-driven competition have altered the characteristics that defined hospitals in 1975 and shaped trends in hospital spending. Table 3–1 shows one of the most tangible effects: between 1975 and 1996, the number of community hospitals dropped from 5,875 to 5,134, while the number of beds declined from more than 1 million to 862,000. At the same time, average occupancy fell from 75 percent to 61.5 percent, and average length of stay from 7.7 to 6.2 days. The average number of beds decreased slightly for public and private nonprofit hospitals, but it increased substantially for investor-owned hospitals from 95 beds to 144 beds.

If we rely on those traditional measures of capacity and utilization, we would conclude that the hospital sector shrank during this time period. But that conclusion is not consonant with underlying trends in hospital spending. In total, spending on hospital services increased sharply, rising from 3.2 percent of national income to 4.7 percent. Thus, the period from 1975 to 1996 was actually one of substantial growth, measured in terms of resource utilization in hospitals.

Although it is more difficult to characterize the typical hospital in the late 1990s than it was in 1975, important unifying characteristics remain:

• Hospitals still offer a wide range of inpatient treatments, but they have moved aggressively into outpatient and other ancillary services.

• Markets remain local.

• Many hospitals now belong to local systems.

• Hospitals and physicians have entered into a wide range of contractual and employment relationships that blur traditional boundaries. There is also some vertical integration with insurers. Fully integrated systems have not, however, become the norm.

• Most hospitals are still nonprofit, and national for-profit chains have made few inroads outside their traditional market niches.

• Hospitals continue to draw the vast majority of their revenues from insurance, and the public share of these revenues has increased.

• Purchasers increasingly use systematic evaluations of cost and quality to select hospitals.

Range of Services

While many hospitals lay claim to having "centers of excellence" in specific clinical areas, most community hospitals continue to treat virtually the full gamut of illnesses. At the same time, community hospitals have complemented their inpatient services with a wide range of outpatient services. The percentage of community hospitals with organized outpatient departments tripled between 1975 and 1988, from 26 percent to 77 percent (American Hospital Association 1976, 1990). By 1996, outpatient services accounted for 31 percent of gross hospital revenue, compared with slightly less than 12 percent in 1975. Between 1992 and 1996 alone, the number of nonemergency hospital outpatient visits surged almost 35 percent, from just under 258 million to almost 347 million (American Hospital Association 1998). The trend was even sharper for small hospitals. Between 1992 and 1996, there was an increase of 53 percent in nonemergency visits to hospitals of fewer than 100 beds, and by 1996, more than 45 percent of the gross revenues at these smaller hospitals came from outpatient services. In percentage terms, while the share of total health spending on hospital inpatient care fell from 30.1 percent in 1980 to 21.9 percent in 1995, the share of total spending on outpatient care more than doubled, rising from 4.5 percent to 9.6 percent (Prospective Payment Assessment Commission 1997).

What explains these trends? Managed care plans and public payers have sought vigorously to reduce inpatient care since the 1980s or earlier. The record suggests, however, that an important effect has been not so much to move services out of the hospital per se, as to move them to another setting within the hospital. A key example has been surgery. Surgery is expensive. For example, the average Medicare reimbursement for an inpatient hernia operation in 1995 exceeded $5,000. The cost of complex procedures can be much higher—for instance, more than $24,000 for a kidney transplant (HCFA 1996). The conventional wisdom holds that costs can be reduced by performing surgery on an outpatient basis whenever possible. In 1984, 28 percent of all surgeries performed at community hospitals were on an outpatient basis. In 1988, only four years later, the share of outpatient surgeries had jumped to 47 percent (American Hospital Association 1990). By 1996, the share of outpatient surgeries had increased to 59 percent; inpatient surgeries were in the minority (American Hospital Association 1998).[12]

The shift from inpatient to outpatient use was accompanied by a general increase in the number of surgeries performed at hospitals. The total number of surgeries at community hospitals grew from 17 million in 1975 to around 21 million in 1987, and in 1996 it was slightly higher than 23 million (American Hospital Association 1976, 1990, 1998).

It is no surprise that hospital-based outpatient care dominated the emerging market for outpatient services in the late 1980s and early 1990s. Economies of scope give hospital-based services an advantage over many free-standing outpatient facilities. Economies of scope were especially important because many of the outpatient services that emerged in the 1980s, including many surgical procedures, were far more complex than traditional outpatient services. For example, an angioplasty may be performed on an outpatient basis, but it is clearly advantageous to have inpatient backup services close at hand should complications arise. Thus, it is striking that in 1996, 62 percent of Medicare spending for outpatient services went for services rendered in hospital outpatient clinics.[13] Although freestanding ambulatory surgery clinics have been growing rapidly, they accounted for only about 3 percent of total Medicare spending on ambulatory services. Moreover, the concentration of volume in hospitals was especially high for complex services such as diagnostic colonoscopies (77.5 percent) and CT scans of the brain and head (86 percent). Even in the area of cataract extractions, where freestanding ambulatory surgery centers have been especially important, the hospital outpatient share was 62 percent (Medicare Payment Advisory Commission 1998).[14]

It is less clear whether the move from hospital-based inpatient care to hospital-based outpatient care was driven by efficiencies or by payment considerations. The hospital bill for inpatient care usually exceeds the bill for comparable outpatient treatment. But differences in charges are not the same as differences in costs. The latter tend to be much smaller, because the bill for inpatient care includes substantial charges for "hotel services," for which hospitals set charges well in excess of the incremental costs. Outpatient treatment conversely shifts the burden of nursing costs from paid hospital staff to unpaid relatives and friends. Because comparisons of charges mask the actual differences in costs, it is conceivable that the incremental cost of inpatient care is lower than that for outpatient care.

Facing potentially substantial differences between charges and economic costs, payers have sought to reduce their own expenses by encouraging outpatient care. Ironically, from a social perspective total medical expenses might be unaffected, or might even increase. Payers have used several strategies to encourage outpatient care. For one, they have followed the lead of HCFA and introduced prospective payment for inpatient care while keeping fee-for-service reimbursements for outpatient care. That can make it more profitable to provide many procedures on an outpatient basis (Drake 1994). At the same time, payers contract with utilization-review agencies that deny claims for inpatient procedures that could have been performed on an outpatient basis.

If it really is less costly to provide inpatient care, then insurers should be able to restructure payments so as to encourage inpatient care while leaving themselves and hospitals better off. For example, insurers could pay a fixed fee per episode of illness, and let providers identify the most efficient setting for care (Dranove and White 1994). The reason why such restructuring of payments has not occurred to any great extent is unclear and is an interesting area for research. Recent changes in Medicare payments for skilled nursing home care represent a move in this direction.

Geographic Markets

The growth of managed care has held out the prospect that purchasers might direct patients to visit out-of-town hospitals to secure substantially lower prices. Indeed, managed care organizations purchase certain highly specialized services, such as organ and bone marrow transplants, in regional markets. By doing so, MCOs can obtain better prices, and perhaps better quality, than if they shopped locally. For example, an MCO might direct a resident of downstate Illinois to a mid-state high-volume "center of excellence" for heart care. In 1975, the same patient might have obtained heart services from a local hospital that cared only for a small number of such patients per year, often at higher costs with lower quality.

To date, there is no systematic evidence of increases attributable to managed care in travel for private patients[15] (Mobley and Frech 1997; White and Morrisey 1998). MCOs still contract for most services with local providers. MCO executives have claimed that hospital networks must include a geographically diverse set of local hospitals to be competitive.[16] Given a choice of local providers, patients continue to prefer the nearest provider, all else being equal. While regional contracting by MCOs for some high-tech services may exist, it has not led to overall increases in patient travel. In part, that may be attributable to increased availability of high-tech services in relatively small markets.

Community Links, Horizontal Integration, and Local Control

Since 1975, there has been growing horizontal integration in the U.S. hospital industry. National investor-owned hospital systems emerged during the 1970s. At their peak in the mid-1980s, for-profit systems such as Hospital Corporation of America (HCA) controlled more than 300 hospitals, and the top five for-profit systems controlled nearly 500 hospitals. (There were no national nonprofit systems to speak of.) Seemingly impressive as that was, it still represented fewer than 10 percent of all general hospitals and an even smaller percentage of beds. For reasons that remain unexplored, the for-profit systems sold off many of the holdings in the late 1980s and early 1990s.

The small, fledgling Columbia system consolidated many of these hospitals into the giant Columbia/HCA system. Unlike previous for-profit systems, Columbia attempted to establish a strong presence in selected local markets, including areas in Florida and Texas. That strategy collapsed, however, after an investigation for Medicare fraud. In the wake of that investigation, Columbia sold off half of its hospitals. Interestingly, it sold off hospitals primarily in urban markets, suggesting that it did not have a viable competitive strategy there. Columbia continues to operate hospitals profitably in markets where it faces little competition.[17]

Although the growth of national chains slowed, local systems, which were mainly nonprofit, grew rapidly beginning in the late 1980s and 1990s. It is difficult to track precisely the growth of local systems. We do know that by 1992, 26 percent of all hospitals reported involvement in local networks (Luke et al. 1995). Moreover, by 1994, 28 percent of all urban hospitals belonged to a "local system" in which two or more hospitals in the same metro area had a common owner.[18] In some markets, such as Chicago's, the vast majority of hospitals are affiliated with one or more local hospitals, leaving few that are completely independent.

Dranove and Shanley (1995) offer several rationales for the emergence of local systems. Local systems can exploit economies of scale in administration, and by consolidating facilities they can reduce production costs as well.

There is mixed evidence on whether local mergers create efficiencies. Dranove and Shanley find no difference in the costs of local systems and independent hospitals. Connor et al. (1997) found that hospital mergers after 1990 generated modest (2 to 3 percent) reductions in costs. Neither study adequately controls for bias that might arise because of self-selection: that is, the possibility that merging hospitals differ from nonmerging hospitals in ways that cannot be measured by the researchers.

Local systems also reduce transactions costs for consumers. Purchasers may prefer the "one-stop shopping" of local systems, and may rely on the system's brand name as an imprimatur of quality. Indeed, an MCO gains credibility with consumers who are concerned about quality by including a well-known local system in its network. Finally, local systems have greater bargaining power with MCOs.

It is interesting to note in the context of these studies that there is also little evidence of a medical arms race (MAR) among hospitals in a managed care environment. Although an MAR may have existed in the 1970s (*see* Robinson and Luft 1985), studies of California, which had high managed care penetration early on, suggest that competitive pressures effectively eliminated the MAR by the mid-1980s (Zwanziger and Melnick 1988). That finding casts doubt on claims that mergers may be a vehicle for eliminating inefficiency from the MAR, at least in markets with high managed care penetration (Kopit and McCann 1988).

Autonomous Medical Staffs and Vertical Integration

Since the mid-1980s, the traditional separations between hospitals and their medical staffs, and between hospitals and insurers, have become increasingly blurred. Hospital employment of physicians, purchase of physician practices, and formation of joint ventures with doctors are all common. In 1996, 20 percent of all community hospitals had at least some physicians on salary; the share was 35 percent for hospitals with 300 beds or more.

During the 1990s, many hospitals and physicians jointly formed Physician Hospital Organizations (PHOs). In 1996 a third of all community hospitals had a PHO, and among hospitals with more than 300 beds, the share with PHOs exceeded 50 percent. PHOs accept capitated payments from insurance companies and deliver a full gamut of medical services. PHOs use a variety of methods to compensate participating physicians. In addition, many hospitals have been involved in setting up Independent Practice Associations, physician management organizations, and a wide variety of other types of arrangements with physicians (American Hospital Association 1998). Finally, there has been widespread discussion of "economic credentialing" of physicians—that is, review of physicians' financial performance as a criterion for staff privileges. While the extent to which this practice has been systematically occurring is unclear, it represents another symptom of the blurring of the lines of authority.

Hospitals have also begun offering their own insurance products. In 1996 some 22 percent of all community hospitals had an ownership interest in an HMO, and 31 percent had an interest in a PPO. Among hospitals with 300 beds or more, some 40 percent had an ownership interest in an HMO and 45 percent in a PPO (American Hospital Association 1998).

Vertical integration appears to be a direct response to managed care. Prominent healthcare analysts, led by Stephen Shortell, have claimed that physician-hospital integration is an effective means to reduce costs and improve quality (Shortell et al. 1996). Not only does this "put everyone on the same page" for cost-containment; it also creates opportunities to develop and implement new clinical guidelines. Providers are eager to integrate as a way of coping with the rapidly changing market, especially where managed care penetration is growing.

Whether or not integration advocates' claims have merit, fundamental problems with vertical integration are only now becoming apparent to healthcare managers. Hospital managers and physicians continue to have their own goals, even when they partner into PHOs or other structures. It has proven difficult to introduce organizational structures, cultures, or incentives that change provider behavior. Integrated organizations are subject to substantial infighting as individuals battle over scarce internal capital. Paul Milgrom and John Roberts (1992) refer to the resulting inefficiencies as *influence costs*. Influence costs manifest themselves in many ways—departments protect unprofitable programs, refuse to partner with other departments, and waste time lobbying for preferential treatment.

It is unclear whether tight, vertically integrated systems represent the wave of the future. Some large integrated systems certainly exist, including the Henry Ford system in Michigan, the Allina Health system in Minnesota, and Sharp Healthcare in California. But most hospitals are not highly vertically integrated. Moreover, the extent of vertical integration in systems is unclear. A 1997 survey is illustrative (Hoechst Marion Roussel 1998). The survey characterized 228 systems as "highly integrated." Hospitals initiated more than 60 percent of these systems, and altogether these systems had formal relationships with 1,584 hospitals. But more than half of these relationships involved arms-length, contractual relationships, as opposed to ownership. While the nature of these contractual relationships bears further investigation, the general pattern suggests that market relationships, rather than direct control, remain a major feature of even highly integrated systems. Furthermore, research by Burns et al. (1998) suggests that the relationship between integrated-system growth and managed care penetration is complex and depends on market structure as well as managed care penetration levels.

Investor-owned versus Nonprofit Organization

Hospitals remain predominantly nonprofit. In 1996, only 759 hospitals were investor-owned. There has recently been an increase in conversions of nonprofit hospitals to for-profit status. Leone and Van Horn (1998) report that between 1991 and 1996, eight for-profit systems purchased eighty-one nonprofit hospitals. More than half of those acquisitions occurred in 1995 and 1996. A number of recent studies have sought to examine factors associated with conversions. Hassett and Hubbard (1998) find that conversions are more frequent in low-income neighborhoods. Barro (1998) also finds a similar pattern. He suggests that one important factor might be the repositioning of hospitals in the marketplace, and he finds that admissions of Medicaid patients fall in these hospitals following conversions.

Critics of conversions worry about the implications for access and quality, and about how investors will deploy the assets of nonprofits—assets that might once have gone to provide community benefit (Claxton et al. 1997; Goddeeris and Weisbrod 1998). In most conversions, the nonprofit assets must be placed in a community trust. But management of the community trust is often intermingled with management of the for-profit hospital, and the trust can use a variety of schemes to return the assets to the investor. For example, the trust may purchase services for the uninsured at prices that vastly exceed incremental costs. State health agencies are concerned about such abuses and are reluctant to approve many conversions. The agency framework we have described suggests that regardless of the disposition of assets in the community trust, state agencies should also assess whether for-profit hospitals will exploit consumer ignorance about quality.

Hospital Revenue Sources

In 1996, as shown in table 3–2, hospitals as a group, including noncommunity hospitals, received just 2.6 percent of revenues directly from consumer out-of-pocket payments. This was down from 8.3 percent in 1975. Hospitals received 62 percent of revenues from public sources, up from 56 percent. While the share of dollars coming from Medicaid actually fell, Medicare's share went from 22 percent in 1975 to 33 percent in 1996 (National Center for Health Statistics 1998). Note that if we consider only community hospitals, the Medicare share is even higher. Private insurance continues to account for about one-third of hospital revenues.

Despite the recent attention given to Medicare managed care, 85 percent of the Medicare population still has traditional indemnity-style coverage, modified only by the PPS. As we discussed earlier, Medicare pays generously for a wide and increasing range of outpatient services— accounting for a major portion of the steady increase in Medicare costs. If new laws further encourage recipients to enroll in managed care, Medicare payments to hospitals may decline.

Two decades ago, a hospital that faced cuts in Medicaid or Medicare payments could potentially compensate by raising prices to private payers. But, as previously discussed, the ability to cost-shift may be sharply constrained by the growth of managed care (Morrisey 1994). Our own research found that when Medicaid payments to California hospitals fell sharply in the late 1980s, the hospitals did not raise prices. Rather, they reduced services provided to Medicaid patients, and some even closed (Dranove and White 1998b).

Quality and Cost Data

Since the early 1980s, major advances have been made in computer technology (such as the growing availability of high-speed, low-cost personal computers), and there has been rapid growth in software applications for hospital use. An increasing number of hospitals have put in place sophisticated internal systems for gathering financial and clinical data.

A growing literature suggests important potential cost savings from these applications (*see* Neumann, Parente, and Paramore 1995). Combined clinical and financial-information systems have also been associated with higher profit margins for hospitals, although the direction of causality is not clear (Parente and Dunbar 1998). Consistent with the use of data in comparison shopping, the provision of detailed financial and utilization information to MCOs also appears to be an important component of contract negotiations.

Even so, it remains a challenge for hospitals to realize the promise of information technology, particularly in linking clinical and financial information (*see* Kleinke 1998). For example, in a recent survey of a representative sample of U.S. hospitals, fewer than half reported having integrated clinical and financial-data systems (Parente and Dunbar 1998). Hospitals are also concerned that managed care is creating large administrative burdens, including information processing, that may offset its potential benefits.

6

The Future of Hospitals

The community hospital has proven to be a surprisingly durable institution in the U.S. healthcare system. Despite dramatic changes in the organization of delivery and finance, it remains the core institutional provider of medical care. In both absolute terms and as a percentage of national income, hospitals are more important than ever. Hospital services still account for more than a third of all healthcare spending, and over time the share of GNP spent on hospital care has grown substantially. Hospitals also remain predominately nonprofit. They continue to play key roles in their local communities, and they are often leading agents for healthcare change.

At the same time, hospitals have significantly repositioned themselves. In 1975, most hospitals were free-standing institutions focused on inpatient care. Today, they increasingly belong to horizontally integrated systems and have expanded their activities to encompass a wide range of outpatient services. There has also been a movement toward vertical integration. The traditional dividing line between hospitals and physicians has blurred. Some hospitals have also become involved in offering insurance products, although fully integrated systems remain relatively rare.

In the context of a shift from patient-driven to payer-driven competition, we have argued that two underlying industry features have combined to maintain the continu-

ing role of the general community hospital as a core provider. The first is economies of scale and scope in providing services, where these economies have been reinforced
by the continuing proliferation of complex technologies.
The second is continuing information problems in coordinating care when moving patients between hospitals, and
between hospitals and other providers.

We have also argued that in the face of growing reliance on payer-driven competition, the changes in hospital organization we have described are consistent with
economies of scale and scope and with information problems. For example, managerial economies of scale and strategic considerations have played a key role in the growth
of horizontal integration in the industry. Increased efficiencies (or at least lower provider costs) and changes in
reimbursement policy have also combined to reduce reliance on inpatient services and to increase reliance on outpatient service within the context of the hospital. Finally,
a blurring of the line between physicians and hospitals is
consistent with a reassessment of the doctor-patient relationship in the face of greater cost pressures and lower
information costs. The same has also been true of relationships between insurers and hospitals.

As illustrated by predictions of the hospital's impend-
ing demise in the early 1980s, speculation about the future of hospitals can be hazardous. Our research suggests,
however, that analysis of the interaction between informational issues and technological change may be a powerful tool for understanding not only the historical
evolution of the hospital industry but the direction in
which it is moving as well.

Technological Change and Information

In the context of the current organization of the healthcare
system, technological change in the production of medical

services could affect the structure of the hospital industry in several ways. First, technological change may increase or decrease the economies of scale and scope associated with centralized production in the hospital. Here, the rate of change, as well as the particular type of change, may be important if hospitals have an advantage in the adoption of new technologies. That is, there may be considerable "first-mover advantage" afforded to hospitals that are early adopters of state-of-the-art care that only subsequently is available elsewhere. Patients will prefer to visit these early adopters, even as the market catches up to them.

Turning to changes in information systems, we have repeatedly emphasized the role of information costs in shaping the organization of healthcare institutions. If new innovations were to lower these costs, a wide range of effects could ensue. If the costs of ensuring continuity of care were to fall, it could become much easier to shift patients between facilities. That could significantly reduce the importance of "option demand" and lower the attractiveness of the traditional general community hospitals, opening the way to a rise in the number of more specialized facilities. Likewise, lower information costs could make it easier to standardize treatments and thus reduce the need for patients to rely on physicians as agents. That could further weaken the case for the traditional division between hospitals and doctors. Finally, consumers and managed care organizations could be greatly facilitated in their ability to shop for care.

We offer several caveats, however, about the effects of changes in information systems. To the extent that information improves, the structure of the way it is gathered may be critical. If information systems develop in such a way that information becomes highly fungible, then not only hospitals but all institutions would move toward decentralization. But if information systems develop in ways that make them operatively organization-specific, then institutions could move toward integration. As the major centralized providers of care, hospitals could well become the hubs of such systems, and their preeminence would increase.

Here, public policy could play an important role. There is a large "public good" aspect to the design of information systems and the creation of industry standards. Public investments that facilitate the development of common standards could move us toward an environment in which information is relatively fungible. In the absence of such standards, we could move in the opposite direction.

Consolidation and Antitrust

A final issue to examine is the general environment in which hospitals operate. As of this writing, there appears to be no immediate likelihood of national healthcare reform. The issue could reemerge, perhaps in response to continuing concerns about access. But in the short run, incremental changes in public policy are more likely to be important. In addition, problems with market-oriented strategies could emerge on their own terms.

Managed care has been predicated on creating more effective competition in healthcare markets. To the extent that such competition generates pressure for integration among hospitals and other providers, it can undermine managed care's future viability as a cost-containment strategy. In our review of the literature on hospital competition, we (Dranove and White 1994) find that managed care functions more effectively in markets with a relatively low hospital concentration. Dranove, Simon, and White (1998) also show that managed care growth is greatest in markets with low hospital concentration. Based, in part, on economic studies such as these, the Federal Trade Commission and the Department of Justice have challenged hospital mergers in smaller metropolitan areas, out of concern that the resulting concentration would limit the ability of managed care purchasers to obtain discounts. Concerns about market power are not limited to hospitals. Physicians are merging into larger groups, joining physician-practice management firms, contemplating unionization, and seeking legislative relief from antitrust laws (Dranove and White 1998a).

Many providers defend consolidation as a necessary response to the growing consolidation of managed care organizations. The recent merger between Aetna and Prudential alarms many providers, who see the combined entity controlling as many as 50 percent of the managed care lives in select markets. A battle is clearly looming in many markets between powerful buyers and powerful sellers.

A key factor in the outcome of this battle will be antitrust policy. If there is no antitrust enforcement in provider markets, then managed care will be stymied as a cost-containment strategy. If there is no enforcement in Managed Care Organization (MCO) markets, then further MCO consolidation seems likely. Implications for providers and consumers could be dire. Providers could find themselves brutally squeezed while, in the absence of market pressure, monopolistic MCOs could withhold their financial gains from consumers. Moreover, in the absence of market pressure, MCOs may fail to innovate and improve quality. Hands-off antitrust policy in both provider and MCO markets could lead to bilateral monopoly with unpredictable consequences.

Tough, even-handed antitrust enforcement in both provider and MCO markets has the potential to preserve the benefits of payer-driven competition. Conversely, failure to maintain competition in these markets has implications well beyond the performance of managed care. For if managed care fails to live up to its potential, in the long run there is likely to be a renewed outcry for a government solution based on regulatory, rather than market, principles.

Medicare

In the near term, perhaps the most important factor affecting the environment in which hospitals operate will be payment policies for public programs. Hospitals still receive nearly half their revenue from Medicare. The Balanced Budget Act of 1997 made important changes in payment formulas for conventional Medicare. It is still too soon to assess the results of this legislation, and we do not attempt to examine its impact here. But a squeeze on hospital profit margins could have far-reaching effects (see Guterman 1999). Hospitals may be further squeezed by an increase in Medicare managed care enrollments. Although there has been considerable turmoil in the Medicare HMO market in the past few years, growth seems likely to continue. If it does, hospitals will have to lower prices to obtain HMO contracts and will also likely see further shifts toward outpatient care. Inner-city and teaching hospitals that relied on Indirect Medical Education (IME) and Disproportionate Share Hospital (DSH) payments could be especially hard hit by those price reductions. That raises issues both about the financing of medical education and about access to care for low-income patients who have traditionally been served by these hospitals.

If managed care comes to dominate Medicare, then the federal government will have a growing interest in maintaining competition and access. HCFA will join MCOs in demanding antitrust vigilance in provider markets. It will also have a powerful interest in maintaining competition in MCO markets. Congress as a result may find itself under pressure from at least three sides—industry players, consumers, and taxpayers. Hospitals, physicians, and other providers will seek greater relief from the strains of competition and pressure from MCOs. MCOs, while advocating competitive provider markets, might also seek protection for themselves. Patients will seek legislation ensuring broad networks and quality assurance. Taxpayers will continue to demand lower Medicare spending growth. Congress will have to strike a balance among these conflicting goals. And the resulting political conflict may further strengthen demands for noncompetitive regulatory reforms.

Notes

1. We use the term integration to imply common owner-ship of assets. Horizontal integration involves the control of assets at the same level of production (such as hospitals), whereas vertical integration involves the control of assets at different levels of production (such as hospitals and physi-cians). There is, of course, a continuum between complete in-dependence and fully functional integration, including joint ventures, strategic alliances, and holding companies. It is beyond the scope of this study to explore this continuum. We focus on integration toward the fully functional, integration end of the spectrum, where there is common ownership of assets and a single entity responsible for setting prices.

2. Arrow (1963) offers a similar explanation for why patients rely so heavily on their physicians. By dint of self-selection, training, and culture, most physicians also have a genuine in-terest in serving the public interest. In this context, while phy-sician practices are typically privately owned, Evans (1984) describes them as "not-only-for-profit" organizations.

3. Note, however, as observed by Starr (1982) and others, that while there were a few prepaid plans, the traditional insurance system benefited from the zealous efforts of orga-nized medicine to exclude them.

4. Children's Hospitals are an important exception. They treat a wide range of illnesses but employ staff especially trained to meet the emotional and physical needs of children and their families.

5. In the past few years, many hospitals have also opened or acquired freestanding clinics and purchased physician practices. That seems to have less to do with scope economies than with a desire by the hospitals to obtain referrals. (Medicare anti-kickback statutes and ethical restrictions on fee-splitting prevent hospitals from simply paying for referrals.)

6. An important exception was physician-owned hospitals.

7. A controversial issue that we do not address here is whether the payment system stimulated the development of cost-increasing technologies (see, for example, Feldstein 1977).

8. Note that while DRGs are partly based on patients' clinical conditions, they also reflect the treatments provided. For example, open-heart–surgery procedures have their own DRGs. Hence, they remain to some degree driven by treatment decisions as well as patients' clinical characteristics.

9. Medicare introduced its Resource Based Relative Value Scale (RBRVS) payment scheme for physicians in 1992, providing a standardized basis for paying physicians. We do not attempt to discuss the implications of this scheme here in any detail, but note that payment continued to be service-based and choice of physician remained patient-driven.

10. We base these figures on our experiences as consultants in a large number of healthcare litigation matters.

11. For example, one of the nation's largest PPOs, First Health (formerly Health Care Compare), started out as a small consulting firm that provided cost comparisons to managed care organizations.

12. For example, hernia operations are largely performed as outpatient procedures; kidney transplants remain an inpatient procedure.

13. That includes physician-practice expenses related to services provided in hospital outpatient departments, but not physician fees.

14. Unfortunately, the data do not distinguish between services provided at the main hospital facility and those provided at satellite facilities.

15. While patients enrolled in MCOs may travel farther for care, that could reflect selection effects. Hence, the relevant question in evaluating effects on travel is whether travel patterns have changed for patients as a group.

16. That is a contentious point in antitrust investigations. Hospitals point out that MCO patients would willingly travel 50 miles or more to out-of-town hospitals to save money. To our knowledge, there are no networks anywhere in the United States that completely exclude local hospitals, so these competing assertions are difficult to evaluate.

17. The other major for-profit chain, Tenet, also tends to operate in smaller markets where there is less competition.

18. We thank Min Guo of the American Hospital Association for providing the data necessary to compute this figure.

References

American Hospital Association. 1976. *Hospital Statistics: 1976 Edition.* Chicago: American Hospital Association.

———. 1990. *Hospital Statistics: 1989–90 Edition.* Chicago: American Hospital Association.

———. 1998. *Hospital Statistics: 1998 Edition.* Chicago: Healthcare InfoSource.

Arnould, R., R. Rich, and W. D. White, eds. 1993. *Competitive Approaches to Health Policy Reform.* Washington, D.C.: Urban Institute Press.

Arrow, K. 1963. "Uncertainty and the Welfare Economics of Medical Care." *American Economic Review* 535: 941–73.

Athey, S., and S. Stern. 1998. "An Empirical Framework for Testing Theories about Complementarity in Organization Design." Unpublished working paper. Cambridge: Massachusetts Institute of Technology.

Barro, J. 1998. "Hospital Conversions to For-Profit Status: Causes and Consequences." Unpublished working paper. Cambridge: Harvard University.

Bartlett, J. 1955. *Familiar Quotations.* 13th ed. New York: Little, Brown.

Burns, R. L., G. Bazzoli, L. Dynan, and D. Wholey. 1998. *Impact of HMO Market Structure on Hospital-based Integrated Delivery Systems.* Unpublished working paper. Philadelphia: Wharton School, University of Pennsylvania.

Claxton, G., J. Feder, D. Shactman, and S. Altman. 1997. "Public Policy Issues in Nonprofit Conversions: An Overview." *Health Affairs* 16: 9–28.

Connor, R., R. Feldman, and B. Dowd. 1997. "The Effects of Market Concentration and Horizontal Mergers on Hospital Costs and Prices." Unpublished working paper. Minneapolis: University of Minnesota.

Cowing, T., A. Holtmann, and S. Powers. 1983. "Hospital Cost Analysis: A Survey and Evaluation of Recent Studies." *Advances in Health Economics and Health Services Research* 4: 257–303.

Drake, D. F. 1994. *Reforming the Health Care Market: An Interpretive Economic History.* Washington, D.C.: Georgetown University Press.

Dranove, D., and R. Ludwick. 1999. "Competition and Pricing by Nonprofit Hospitals: A Reassessment of Lynk's Analysis." *Journal of Health Economics* 18: 87–98.

Dranove, D., and M. Satterthwaite. Forthcoming. "Industrial Organization of Health Care." In J. Newhouse, ed., *The Handbook of Health Economics.* New York: Elsevier.

———. 1992. "Monopolistic Competition When Price and Quality Are Not Perfectly Observable." *RAND Journal of Economics* 23: 518–34.

Dranove, D., and M. Shanley. 1995. "Cost Reductions or Reputation Enhancement as Motives for Mergers: The Logic of Multihospital Systems." *Strategic Management Journal* 16: 55–74.

Dranove, D., M. Shanley, and C. J. Simon. 1992. "Is Hospital Competition Wasteful?" *RAND Journal of Economics* 23: 247–62.

Dranove, D., M. Shanley, and W. D. White. 1993. "Price and Concentration in Hospital Markets: The Switch from Patient-driven to Payor-driven Competition." *Journal of Law and Economics* 36: 179–204.

Dranove, D., C. J. Simon, and W. D. White. 1998. "Determinants of Managed Care Penetration." *Journal of Health Economics* 17: 729–46.

Dranove, D., and W. D. White. 1987. "Agency and the Organization of Health Care Delivery." *Inquiry* 24: 405–15.

———. 1994. "Recent Theory and Evidence on Competition in Hospital Markets." *Journal of Economics and Management Strategy* 3: 169–209.

———. 1996. "Specialization, Option Demand, and the Pricing of Medical Services." *Journal of Economics and Management Strategy* 5: 277–306.

———. 1998a. "Emerging Issues in the Antitrust Definition of Healthcare Markets." *Health Economics* 7:167–70.

———. 1998b. "Medicaid Dependent Hospitals and Their Patients: How Have They Fared?" *Health Services Research* 33: 163–86.

Dranove, D., W. D. White, and L. Wu. 1993. "Segmentation in Local Hospital Markets." *Medical Care* 31: 52–64.

Emmons, D., and C. J. Simon. 1996. "Managed Care: Evolving Contractual Arrangements." In *Socioeconomic Characteristics of Medical Practice 1996*. Chicago: American Medical Association.

Ermann, D., and J. Gabel. 1984. "Multihospital Systems: Issues and Empirical Findings." *Health Affairs* 3: 50–64.

Evans, R. G. 1984. *Strained Mercy: The Economics of Canadian Health Care*. Toronto: Butterworths.

Feldstein, M. S. 1977. "The High Cost of Hospitals—and What to Do about It." *The Public Interest* 48: 40–54.

Fishman, L., and J. Bentley. 1997. "The Evolution of Support for Safety-Net Hospitals." *Health Affairs* 16: 30–47.

Friedman, B. 1988. *Hospital Restructuring under PPS and Competitive Pressures*. Unpublished working paper. Chicago: Hospital Research and Educational Trust.

Friedman, B. and M. Pauly. 1981. "Cost Functions for a Service Firm with Variable Quality and Stochastic Demand: The Case of Hospitals." *Review of Economics and Statistics* 63: 620–24.

Fuchs, V. 1983. *Who Shall Live?* New York: Basic Books.

Goddeeris, J., and B. Weisbrod. 1998. "Conversion from Nonprofit to For-Profit Legal Status: Why Does It Happen and Should Anyone Care?" *Journal of Policy Analysis and Management* 17: 215–33.

Goldsmith, J. C. 1980. "The Health Care Market: Can Hospitals Survive?" *Harvard Business Review* 58 (September–October): 100–112.

———. 1981. *Can Hospitals Survive? The New Competitive Health Care Market.* Homework, Ill.: Dow Jones-Irwin.

Guterman, S. 1999. "The Balanced Budget Act of 1997: What Are the Implications for Hospitals?" Unpublished working paper. Washington D.C.: Urban Institute.

Hansmann, H. 1980. "The Role of Nonprofit Enterprise." *Yale Law Journal* 89: 835–901.

Harris, J. 1977. "The Internal Organization of Hospitals." *Bell Journal of Economics* 8: 467–82.

Hassett, K., and R. Hubbard. 1998. "How Entrepreneurial Are Not-for-Profit Hospitals?" Unpublished working paper. Washington, D.C.: American Enterprise Institute.

Havighurst, C. C. 1988. "The Questionable Cost-Containment Record of Commercial Health Insurers." In H. E. Frech III, ed., *Health Care in America.* San Francisco: Pacific Research Institute for Public Policy.

Health Care Financing Administration. 1996. Table: "Bureau of Data Management and Strategy from the 100 Percent Medpar Inpatient Hospital Fiscal Year 1995, Short Stay by State." (http://www.hcfa.gov/stats/ss95both.txt.)

Herzlinger, R. 1997. *Market-driven Health Care.* Reading, Mass.: Addison-Wesley.

Hoechst Marion Roussel. 1998. *Managed Care Digest Series 1998: Integrated Health Systems Digest.* Kansas City, Mo.: Hoechst Marion Roussel.

Keeler, E. B., G. Melnick, and J. Zwanziger. 1999. "The Changing Effects of Competition on Non-Profit and For-Profit Hospital Pricing Behavior." *Journal of Health Economics* 18: 69–86.

Kleinke, J. D. 1998. "Release 0.0: Clinical Information Technology in the Real World." *Health Affairs* 17: 23–38.

Kopit, W., and R. McCann. 1988. "Towards a Definitive Anti-Trust Standard for Nonprofit Hospital Mergers." *Journal of Health Politics, Policy and Law* 13: 83–97.

Leone, A. J., and R. L. Van Horn. 1998. "Agency Problems in Corporate Control Transactions and Not-For-Profit Organizations: Evidence from the Healthcare Industry." Unpublished working paper. Rochester: William E. Simon Graduate School of Business Administration, University of Rochester.

Luke, R., Y. Ozcan, and P. Olden. 1995. "Local Markets and Systems: Hospital Consolidations in Metropolitan Areas." *Health Services Research* 30: 555–76.

Lynk, W. 1995. "The Creation of Economic Efficiencies in Hospital Mergers." *Journal of Health Economics* 14: 507–610.

———. 1996. "Nonprofit Hospital Mergers and the Exercise of Market Power." *Journal of Law and Economics* 38: 437–61.

Marmor, T. R., M. Schlesinger, and R. Smithey. 1986. "A New Look at Nonprofits: Health Care Policy in a Competitive Age." *Yale Journal of Regulation* 3: 313–49.

McGuirk, M., and F. Porell. 1984. "Spatial Patterns of Hospital Utilization: The Impact of Time and Distance." *Inquiry* 21: 84–95.

Mechanic, D. 1998. "The Functions and Limitations of Trust in the Provision of Medical Care." Unpublished working paper. New Brunswick, N.J.: Rutgers University.

Medicare Payment Advisory Commission. 1998. *Report to the Congress: Context for a Changing Medicare Program, June 1998.* Washington, D.C.: Medicare Payment Advisory Commission.

Milgrom, P., and J. Roberts. 1992. *Economics, Organization and Management.* Englewood Cliffs, N.J.: Prentice Hall.

Milkenson, M. 1997. *Demanding Medical Excellence.* Chicago: University of Chicago Press.

Mobley, L., and H. E. Frech III. 1997. "Managed Care, Distance Traveled, and Hospital Market Definition: An Exploratory Analysis." Unpublished working paper. Oakland, Calif.: Department of Economics, Oakland University.

Morrisey, M. 1994. *Cost Shifting in Health Care: Separating Evidence from Rhetoric.* Washington, D.C.: AEI Press.

Morrisey, M., F. A. Sloan, and J. Valvona. 1988. "Geographic Markets for Hospital Care." *Law and Contemporary Problems* 51: 165–94.

National Center for Health Statistics. 1988. *Health, United States 1988.* DHHS Publication (PHS) 89-1232.

———. 1998. *Health, United States 1998.* DHHS Publication (PHS) 98-1232.

Neumann, P., S. T. Parente, and L. C. Paramore. 1995. "Potential Savings from Using Information Technology Applications in Health Care in the United States." *International Journal of Technology Assessment in Health Care* 12: 425–35.

Newhouse, J. P. 1992. "Medical Care Costs: How Much Welfare Loss?" *Journal of Economic Perspectives* 6: 3–21.

Noether, M. 1988. "Competition among Hospitals." *Journal of Health Economics* 7: 259–84.

Norton, E., and D. Staiger. 1994. "How Hospital Ownership Affects Access to Care for the Uninsured." *RAND Journal of Economics* 25: 171–85.

Parente, S., and J. Dunbar. 1998. "Does Information Technology Improve the Financial Performance of U.S. Hospitals?" Unpublished working paper. Bethesda, Md.: Project HOPE.

Phelps, C. , and C. Mooney. 1993. "Variations in Medical Practice Use: Causes and Consequences." In R. Arnould, R. Rich, and W. D. White, eds., *Competitive Approaches to Health Policy Reform*. Washington, D.C.: Urban Institute Press.

Prospective Payment Assessment Commission (ProPAC). 1997. *Medicare and the American Health Care System: Report to the Congress, June 1997*. Washington, D.C.: Prospective Payment Assessment Commission.

Robinson, J., and H. Luft. 1985. "The Impact of Hospital Market Structure on Patient Volume, Average Length of Stay, and the Cost of Care." *Journal of Health Economics* 4: 333–56.

Shleifer, A. 1985. "A Theory of Yardstick Competition." *RAND Journal of Economics* 16: 319–27.

Shortell, S., R. Gillies, D. Anderson, K. Erickson, and J. Mitchell. 1996. *Remaking Health Care in America: Building Organized Delivery Systems*. San Francisco: Jossey Bass.

Sloan, F., G. Picone, D. Taylor, and S. Chou. 1998. "Hospital Ownership and Cost and Quality of Care: Is There a Dime's Worth of Difference?" Unpublished working paper. Durham, N.C.: Duke University.

Smith, D. 1992. *Paying for Medicare: The Politics of Reform*. New York: Aldine De Gruyter.

Starr, Paul. 1982. *The Social Transformation of American Medicine*. New York: Basic Books.

Stevens, R. 1971. *American Medicine and the Public Interest*. New Haven, Conn.: Yale University Press.

———. 1989. *In Sickness and in Wealth: American Hospitals in the Twentieth Century*. New York: Basic Books.

Town, R., and G. Vistnes. 1997. "Hospital Competition in HMO Networks: An Empirical Analysis of Hospital Pricing Behavior." Unpublished working paper. Irvine: University of California.

U.S. Bureau of the Census. 1975. *Historical Statistics of the United States, Colonial Times to 1970, Bicentennial Edition, Part 1.* Washington, D.C.

Weisbrod, B. 1988. *The Nonprofit Economy.* Cambridge, Mass.: Harvard University Press.

———. 1989. "Rewarding Performance That Is Hard to Measure: The Private Non-Profit Sector." *Science* 244: 541–46.

———. 1991. "The Health Care Quadrilemma: An Essay on Technological Change, Insurance, Quality of Care, and Cost Containment." *Journal of Economic Literature* 29: 523–52.

White, W. D. 1979. *Public Health and Private Gain: The Economics of Licensing Clinical Laboratory Personnel.* New York: Maaroufa Press/Routledge.

———. 1982. "The American Hospital Industry since 1900: A Short History." In R. Scheffler and L. Rossiter, eds., *Advances in Health Services Research*, vol. 3. Greenwich, Conn.: JAI Press.

———. 1990. "The 'Corporatization' of U.S. Hospitals: What Can We Learn from the Nineteenth-Century Industrial Experience?" *International Journal of Health Services* 20: 85–113.

White, W. D., and M. Morrisey. 1998. "Are Patients Traveling Further?" *International Journal of the Economics of Business* 5: 203–21.

Zwanziger, J., and G. A. Melnick. 1988. "The Effects of Hospital Competition and the Medicare PPS Program on Hospital Behavior in California." *Journal of Health Economics* 7: 301–20.

About the Authors

DAVID DRANOVE is the Richard Paget Distinguished Professor of Management and Strategy at Northwestern University's Kellogg Graduate School of Management. He is also a professor of health services management. He has a Ph.D. in business economics from Stanford University. Professor Dranove's research focuses on problems in industrial organization and business strategy, with an emphasis on the healthcare industry. He received the John Thompson Prize in 1993 from AUPHA and the Marriott Corporation Health Care Services Faculty Publication of the Year Award in 1993 and 1996.

WILLIAM D. WHITE is an associate professor of public health and the head of the Health Management Program in the Department of Epidemiology and Public Health at the Yale University School of Medicine. He received his Ph.D. from Harvard University. His primary area of interest is health economics, with particular focus on the question of how competition is working in healthcare markets.

The authors were jointly awarded the National Institute for Health Care Management's Fifth Annual Health Care Research Award in 1998. In 1999 they received the Article of the Year Award from the Association for Health Services Research.

A NOTE ON THE BOOK

This book was edited by Cheryl Weissman
of the Publications Staff of the
American Enterprise Institute.
The text was set in New Century Schoolbook.
Electronic Quill of Silver Spring,
Maryland, set the type, and
Edwards Brothers of Lillington,
North Carolina, printed and bound the book,
using permanent acid-free paper.

The AEI Press is the publisher for the American Enterprise Institute for Public Policy Research, 1150 17th Street, N.W., Washington, D.C. 20036; *Christopher DeMuth,* publisher; *James Morris,* director; *Ann Petty,* editor; *Leigh Tripoli,* editor; *Cheryl Weissman,* editor; *Kenneth Krattenmaker,* art director and production manager; *Jean-Marie Navetta,* production assistant.